The Simplified Guide to *Permanent* Fat Loss:

Results <u>Without</u> Lifestyle Restriction

Daniel McConnell

Text copyright © 2018 Daniel McConnell
All Rights Reserved

Table of Contents

Introduction

This book is for anybody who wants to make changes to their body but doesn't know exactly what to do. I've been there, and I know how incredibly frustrating it is. These days, many things are easier because of the internet. Almost anybody can have access to any piece of information they want. You can learn so much about so many topics. Unfortunately, because of monetary incentives, the internet has been completely polluted with misinformation and lies about fitness and fat loss.

When I started my weight-loss journey a few years ago, I was considered overweight or obese by every metric. I was so unhappy with myself, and I had no idea what to do. Well, I knew that I had to be more active, and that I had to change the way I ate, but I didn't know *specifically* what to do. Should I eat carbs? Should I not eat carbs? What kind of cardio should I do? And how often? Does meal timing matter? And what about hormones? Does my body purposely make changes to sabotage all my efforts? Are my efforts even worth it? Or am I going to sacrifice everything I enjoy for nothing?

Making changes to your lifestyle and body are very emotional tasks. Fitness marketing is designed to take advantage of that fact. People want you to think that the one thing standing between you and the fitness cover model is one *little trick* that only they know. In addition, they use half-truths to make their claims sound more scientific or logical. In this book, I will cover what is fact and what is fiction. My methods are based on the highest quality and most comprehensive research. I don't teach anything that I don't personally use to achieve my goals. I can proudly say that once I finally figured it out, I was able to lose over 60 pounds and decrease my body fat by over 25%. For the first time in my entire life, I could see my abs. What an incredible feeling. Fast-forward a few years and now I maintain a similar physique on minimal effort and even less lifestyle restriction. And that's exactly what I am going to teach you how to do.

This book will not only teach you the concepts you need to understand about fat loss, but it will also give you the tools you need to create your own plan and achieve and maintain your goals without sacrificing everything you enjoy.

Chapter 1: The Basics

To start, it's important to understand some basics about the human body. Part of this journey is learning how the body works so that you can identify misinformation as you stumble across it. Believe me, it's all over the place. The truth can be harder to find than the myths. You don't need to be an expert in biology to lose fat. But, losing fat is a biological process. Body-fat is considered an organ. It has its own blood vessels, nerve cells, and immune cells. It produces vital hormones and serves as a connective tissue. It is essential for health, and yet, too much of it is strongly correlated with several deadly diseases and conditions. If you want to understand how to lose it, you have to understand why it's there.

Energy

Our bodies need energy to carry out processes and movements to survive. When we eat food, that food gets broken down and used to produce energy. In our bodies, energy comes in the form of a chemical called ATP. ATP requires energy to hold its molecular structure together. Our bodies break down that chemical bond to release and use that energy. This energy is used for everything: organ function, digestion, muscle contractions, body heat, etc. This energy is measured in *calories*. So, ATP is the bodies universal form of energy, and calories are the universal measurement of that energy. When you look at a food label and read the calorie content, you are reading how much energy that food item contains.

Macronutrients

The food you eat is composed of four different compounds that supply energy. These are referred to as macronutrients. They differ based on their chemical structure. The four macronutrients are proteins, carbohydrates, fats, and alcohol. Based on the way our bodies break them down, each one has a different amount of energy per gram. Protein contains four calories per gram. Carbohydrates also contain four calories per gram. Alcohol contains seven calories per gram. Fat contains nine calories per gram.

Often times these categories are broken down even further to sub-categories. For example, there are simple and complex carbohydrates. There are complete and incomplete proteins. There are also several types of fat. In reality, these distinctions aren't very important for fat loss. Food also contains micronutrients, which are compounds that don't contain energy but are vital for overall health. Micronutrients include vitamins, minerals, and phytochemicals such as antioxidants.

The food you eat contains some ratio of the three macronutrients (excluding alcohol). Some foods are very high in one macronutrient and very low in others, but it's very rare to find a food item that doesn't have at least a small portion of all three. Each macronutrient also plays a unique role in the body. Protein helps rebuild tissue. Fat is a precursor to many hormones and is an important energy source. Carbohydrates provide energy for intense exercise and also provide many micronutrients and fiber.

Chapter 2: Digestion, Storage, and Metabolism

In addition to containing different amounts of energy, each macronutrient has a unique way of getting digested, stored, and burned for energy. This information may be completely new to you. It may also be a bit much if you don't enjoy science. I recommend trying to retain as much as possible without worrying about every little detail. With that being said, I have found that many clients have better adherence to their plan the more that they understand the science behind what they're doing. This book will teach you the how, the why, and the what, about fat loss. But before you can learn *what* to do, you have to learn the *how* and *why*.

Fat

Let's start with dietary fat. When fat is consumed, it comes in the form of a *triacylglyceride,* which is just a fancy name for its chemical structure. It is composed of three fatty acids attached to a glycerol backbone. When triacylglycerides get ingested, they must be broken down to be absorbed. Enzymes release the fatty acids from the glycerol, and then they are absorbed by the intestines. From there, they reform back into a triacylglyceride and get packaged into a giant glob of fat called a *chylomicron*. This happens because they are *hydrophobic,* meaning they want to avoid water. These giant globs enter the lymphatic system, and then eventually reach the blood stream. Once they become part of circulation, their contents have two possible destinations: they can be stored for later use or burned for energy.

For the portion that gets stored, they must be broken down once more. The fatty acids cross the membrane of a fat cell, called an *adipocyte,* where they get stored. The average adult has about 30 billion fat cells which are packed with triacylglycerides, and that's what body fat is. The other portion that gets burned for energy must also be broken down. The fatty acids enter a cell where they go through a process to create ATP. Either way, the remaining glycerol portion circulates through the blood, and is either used to form new triacylglyceride from free fatty acids or it can travel to the liver and be converted to glucose by a process called *gluconeogenesis*. So, fat can actually be converted to sugar in the right conditions.

Carbohydrates

Carbohydrates are just a specific type of organic molecule. They are bit less complex than fat. As mentioned earlier, there are two main types:

Simple and complex. Simple carbohydrates are also called sugars. They include glucose, fructose, sucrose, lactose, and more. Complex carbohydrates are also called starches and are formed when multiple glucose molecules combine. Glucose is one of the most important energy sources for the body. The brain and nervous system rely heavily on glucose to produce ATP. Most dietary carbohydrates are either broken down into glucose or converted into glucose by the liver. This glucose enters the bloodstream and becomes what is known as "blood sugar". Stable blood sugar is vital for proper metabolic function. A relatively normal amount of carbohydrate intake results in stable blood sugar. The ingestion of high levels of simple carbohydrates can result in the spike of blood sugar, which triggers a release of insulin. Insulin is simply a hormone the regulates the uptake of glucose by cells.

The fate of blood glucose ultimately depends on several factors including blood glucose levels, overall calorie intake, overall dietary carbohydrate intake, and more. Similar to how triacylglyceride are stored in fat cells, glucose can be stored for later use in both muscle tissue and in the liver. Stored glucose is called *glycogen and* can be formed by linking thousands of glucose molecules in those tissues. The average adult can store about 75-100 grams of glycogen in the liver and about 12 grams in every kilogram of muscle tissue. This is generally about 350-400 grams, which means that the average adult can store between 1,700 and 2,000 calories worth of glucose in the liver and muscles. Due to its chemical structure, every gram of glycogen that gets stored is accompanied by three grams of water. This means that changes in carbohydrate intake can affect your body weight by affecting the amount of water stored in your body. This is important to remember. The conversion of dietary carbohydrate into fat is possible via a process called *de novo lipogenesis*. However, this typically only takes place when carbohydrate and calorie intake are both excessive, and when glycogen storages are full.

Protein

Protein plays the key role of supporting the growth and repair of tissues. Proteins are composed of amino acids, of which there are twenty. Nine of the twenty amino acids are considered essential, meaning they must be obtained through dietary means. The remaining eleven are considered non-essential, not because they aren't important, but rather because they can be produced by the body. Protein digestion is also a bit less complex than fat digestion. The body breaks down dietary proteins into amino acids, which enter the blood stream through the intestines. From there, the amino acids can be used to reform proteins, rebuild tissue, or form enzymes. They can also be transported to the liver where *gluconeogenic* amino acids can be converted into glucose, and *ketogenic* amino acids can be used either for energy production or converted into fat. Thirteen amino acids are exclusively gluconeogenic, five are both gluconeogenic and ketogenic, and the remaining two are exclusively ketogenic. Protein can also be formed from carbohydrates and fats, but this only takes place when the body has excess amino acids from which the nitrogen component may be used.

Alcohol

For our purposes, we won't go into the details of alcohol digestion. Alcohol does not get stored for later use like the other macronutrients because the body wants to get rid of it as fast as possible. The important thing to remember about alcohol is that does contain seven calories per gram, making it more calorie-dense than both carbohydrates and proteins.

As we covered, each of the three main macronutrients can be chemically converted into another macronutrient or a substrate of another macronutrient. This is an important fact. The body compensates for restrictive diets. Cutting out carbohydrates doesn't mean that no glucose exists in the body. Cutting out fat does not mean that nothing you eat can be stored as fat. Each macronutrient plays its own role, and its much easier to fit each one into your nutrition plan than to force your body to create them.

Chapter 3: Metabolism

Now that you have a solid understanding of how each macronutrient gets stored and used within the body, let's cover your body's metabolism and how it creates energy with those molecules.

Metabolism is a term that is used all the time, yet it seemed to be often misused and misunderstood. Metabolism refers to the sum of all chemical processes essential for life. It is a very complicated process that includes a multitude of chemical reactions. This process is constant. The human body is always in a state of breaking down while simultaneously in a state of building up. Fat is always being stored and always being burned. Muscle is always being broken down and always being synthesized. The net balance is what determines your body composition. Metabolic *rate* refers to the rate at which your body utilizes energy. Essentially, it's the number of calories you burn, usually measured on a daily basis. The total number of calories you burn every day is also called your Total Daily Energy Expenditure (TDEE). There are several components that make up your TDEE. Let's start with Resting Metabolic Rate (RMR), sometimes referred to as your basal metabolic rate. This term refers to the number of calories you burn simply by being alive. If you were to lay still in a bed all day, you would still burn these calories. They come from the energy your body expends behind the scenes performing vital bodily functions. This makes up about 70% of your TDEE. Your RMR is determined by several factors, mainly your genetics and your body composition. More on that later. Next is Non-Exercise Activity Thermogenesis (NEAT). This term is defined differently by different fitness professionals and researchers, but I like to define it as the sum of both the conscious and subconscious activity that could not be considered exercise. Essentially, it refers to the energy you expend doing your daily activities: getting out of bed, getting dressed, talking, cooking, cleaning, fidgeting, etc. The reason I mentioned both conscious and subconscious activity is that they respond to dieting differently. This phenomenon will be covered in greater depth later on. Alongside NEAT, there's Exercise-Activity Thermogenesis (EAT). This is the energy that you expend from exercise. NEAT and EAT typically make up about 20% of total daily energy expenditure. Surprisingly, NEAT generally makes up a greater portion of your energy expenditure than EAT. Finally, there is the Thermic Effect of Food (TEF), which is the energy required to digest the food you eat. So, you eat food that contains energy, but your body requires energy to break down that food to get energy out of it. TEF is generally the remaining 10% of TDEE.

Time for a brief recap. The total number of calories you burn every day is called your total daily energy expenditure (TDEE), and it is determined by the number of calories your body uses to perform bodily functions, to break down food, to perform daily tasks, and to exercise. **Most of the energy you burn every day comes from your resting metabolic rate, and that amount is determined primarily by your genetics and by your body composition.** The statement you just read is very important. Hopefully you noticed that the average person burns twice as many calories just from bodily functions than they burn from all their daily activities and exercise combined. One reason why so many people fail is that they focus solely on one component of TDEE rather than the entire equation. The good news is that each of the four components can be manipulated or influenced, and the coming chapters will teach you how to do so.

Energy Systems

Now that you are familiar with the components of your metabolic rate, let's cover your body's different energy systems. As you already know, each macronutrient is used to make ATP. These molecules are generally not used exclusively. They contribute to energy production in ratios, based on certain factors. There are two main states that your body can be in: aerobic and anaerobic. Aerobic means that your oxygen intake is equal to the amount of oxygen your body needs. This is the state you are in the majority of the time. You become anaerobic when you need more oxygen than you're taking in, which happens during intense exercise. Energy production happens on a spectrum similar to human activity. Our activity ranges from sleeping, to sitting on our butts doing nothing, to walking, to maximum intensity exercise. Have you ever wondered why we are able to perform easier or less intense activities for much longer than intense activities? It's not simply because they are easier; it has to do with how our bodies make energy. At rest, we have enough oxygen, and our bodies use aerobic metabolism to make energy. In this state, we burn roughly 60-75% fat, 20-35% carbohydrates, and about 5% protein. As our activity becomes more intense, that ratio shifts to burning less fat and more carbohydrates. This is where the "fat burning zone" myth came about. It's better to burn a higher percentage of fat, right? Actually, that's not the case. At higher intensities you burn more overall calories, which means you burn more fat and more carbohydrates. Burning more carbohydrates means that future carbohydrate intake will be more likely to replace those carbohydrates rather than get stored as fat, which is why burning more calories overall is a win-win. As the intensity of the activity increases, you will eventually hit a point where oxygen demand exceeds oxygen intake. This is where you become anaerobic, and your body will begin to burn exclusively carbohydrates, or glucose. The process of creating ATP anaerobically is called *anerobic glycolysis*. It makes energy very fast, but this comes at a price. This system causes a buildup of a chemical called lactic acid, which shuts the system down once it reaches a certain concentration. Lactic acid is what causes the burning sensation in your muscles during exercise. Once the system shuts down, you'll be forced to decrease your intensity until you can take in enough oxygen and buffer the lactic acid.

It is physically impossible to remain anaerobic for more than a few minutes, even for elite athletes. This means that your body uses aerobic systems, and therefore fat, as fuel most of the time. If you've ever heard someone talk about fat burning as though it has to be "activated" by some supplement or some special exercise or dieting technique, just know that this is not the case and now you know why!

Chapter 4: Why Calories Are Key

Now that you understand what the macronutrients are, what roles they play, the components of your metabolism, and your body's energy systems, let's talk about why calories are the most important factor in regard to losing fat.

This seems to be the area where most fitness and dieting myths arise. People are very enthusiastic about certain diets that focus on aspects other than calorie intake. As much as it frustrates me, I understand why. Weight loss can be very emotional. Food can be emotional. Some diets are based on health, some diets are based on moral beliefs. With emotional subjects, people become very attached to their beliefs. They may see success from one dieting method and become convinced that there is no other way, when in reality there probably is.

Most fad diets that have gained popularity over the years are restrictive in nature. They focus on the idea that (fill in the blank) is what you should *not* eat. The most confusing part is that the most enthusiastic people fall on opposite sides on the spectrum. The people who say that carbohydrates are the enemy as just as convincing as the people who say you should only eat carbs. Those who push low-carb diets have just as many scientific-sounding reasons as those who push low-fat diets.

The reason that so many opposing diets have followers and promoters is that they've all seen at least some level of short-term success. People *have* lost weight on them, plain and simple. But it's not because they each have some magic formula that works for some and not for others. Rather, it's because their unnecessarily restrictive nature indirectly led to lower calorie intake and short-term results for some of their followers. If you follow a low-carb diet, you end up cutting out an entire macronutrient. It would be pretty difficult to do so without lowering calorie intake. The same can be said for low-fat diets, as well as Keto, Paleo, vegan, carnivore and every other fad-diet option out there. This does *not* mean that these diets are optimal.

In reality, the most recent and well-structured studies have shown that when calorie and protein intake are equated, there is <u>zero</u> difference in fat loss between high-fat/low-carb and high-carb/low-fat diets. Even more surprising is that the same holds true even when the high-carbohydrate groups ate high levels of simple or processed sugars. This is also true even when the high-fat diets could be considered ketogenic, which is a fad diet that has been growing in popularity. There has also consistently been no difference between health markers such as resting metabolic rate, insulin sensitivity, preservation of muscle mass, or even blood markets such as LDL, HDL, or triglycerides. It turns out that the process of losing excess bodyfat has such a positive impact on health that it outweighs eating what some would consider to be "unhealthy" foods.

It's important to understand that "healthy" is a relative term. How many times have you heard someone say, "I don't understand why I'm not losing weight I've been eating healthy for a month!". This is because you can eat "healthy" foods and still consume far too many calories. As more and more research is done, we are starting to see that there really is no such thing as a healthy or unhealthy food item. Every food item is different. Some foods contain a lot of energy, some foods contain less. Some foods contain a lot of vitamins and minerals, some contain very little. When determining if something is "healthy", it really depends on how much energy your body needs, which micronutrients your body needs, and what other foods you're consuming in your diet. There are tons of food items that are widely regarded as being extremely healthy, that you should not simply start snacking on unless you are replacing another food item and properly taking everything into account. A recent study comparing calorie-equated diets composed of different foods found that 95-100% of the health benefits came strictly from the process of losing excess weight rather than the composition of the diet. The bottom line is that we now know beyond any shadow of a doubt that it doesn't matter what you restrict, or what you cut out, or what you don't cut out of your diet; if you burn more calories than you take in, you <u>will</u> lose fat, and there are tons of health benefits associated with that.

The state of burning more calories than you take in over time is called a *caloric deficit*. Before going any farther, I want you to understand the science behind how a negative energy balance, or a caloric deficit, actually causes fat loss. After this section, you should have no doubt in your mind that you're doing the right thing when you follow the plan laid out in the coming chapters. Let's start with the distinction between weight loss and fat loss. They are not the same, but they are correlated. As you enter a caloric deficit, the net outputs from metabolism outweigh the inputs. Your body is now using more than it is storing. The question is, what exactly is it using more of? Your body will do everything it possibly can to preserve blood glucose levels, we well as glycogen since it is a backup source for blood glucose and very important for intense movements. Since blood glucose and stored glycogen are preserved, this only leaves two remaining components for weight loss. The first is fat, and the second is lean body mass. Lean body mass simply refers to anything that isn't fat: bone, muscles, organs, blood, water, etc. As you lose weight, you will lose a very small portion from fluids and other non-muscle components of lean body mass, but let's put that aside for now. This essentially leaves two options: bodyfat and muscle.

Obviously, the goal is to maintain as much muscle as possible and maximize the amount of fat being lost. The amount of fat lost from a calorie deficit really depends on what is happening with muscle tissue. Recall from the chapter on metabolism that muscle tissue is a constant flux on amino acids. In a calorie deficit, the amount of amino acids leaving the muscle will most likely outweigh the amount entering the muscle. This is because the overall level of substrates from food intake is lower, and the body will send gluconeogenic amino acids to the liver to be converted to glucose in order to help preserve blood glucose levels. This is why the studies comparing fat loss between different diets made sure that *both* calories and protein were equated.

Research shows us that people who lose weight through dieting alone lose roughly 60% fat and 40% muscle. This is not ideal, but it is still mostly fat. If you add to the equation sufficient protein intake, and consistent resistance training, the numbers look more like 80% fat and 20% muscle. Resistance training causes the body to put greater emphasis on the remodeling of muscle tissue and thus more amino acids will be used for that process. Adequate protein intake will result in a smaller flux of amino acids out of the muscle. Even better news is that if you're relatively new to resistance training, or have taken a long break from it, there is a good chance you will preserve a much higher amount of muscle mass, resulting in a loss of nearly 100% bodyfat. By properly manipulating those variables, a calorie deficit will result in fat loss simply because it *must* result in a loss of body-mass, and your body preserves everything else.

I can't stress enough how important it is to understand that a calorie deficit *by definition* will cause weight loss. This fact is supported by the first law of thermodynamics. Your body is converting matter into energy and expending more than it is storing. Regardless, there are still people out there trying to debunk this fact. They would have as much success debunking the theory of gravity. Many people make the mistake of estimating their calorie intake or calorie expenditure wrong, and then believing that a calorie deficit did not work for them, which is not the case. It was simply a discrepancy between the estimated numbers and reality. Many people also claim that calories don't matter if certain hormone levels are out of balance. Hormones actually respond to energy balance, rather than the other way around. So yes, hormones do have an effect, but they simply effect either side of the energy balance equation through effecting your metabolic rate or indirectly effecting your energy intake through hunger signals. A perfect example of this is insulin. Many people say that it is impossible to lose fat, even in a calorie deficit, if you have high insulin levels. In reality, a calorie deficit by itself decreases insulin levels and increases insulin sensitivity. Hormones have an effect, but they are secondary to the most important aspect which will always be your caloric balance.

Chapter 5: Building Your Fat Loss Roadmap

You've now learned some critical concepts and understand what the main goal should be when trying to lose fat. One thing I've noticed in the fitness world is that things are either made to be extremely complex or they are over-simplified. There isn't much of a middle ground. There is the crowd that basically says you have to eat certain foods at a certain time, or your hormones will do something to make your body cling to fat. Then there's the crowd that says, "just eat less". In reality, the best plan is one that gives you the flexibility to enjoy life but also has a detailed list of steps that must be followed accurately. That's exactly what this roadmap will be. It's not a quick fix. Rather, it's a compilation of tools that you can use for the rest of your life to maintain a physique and lifestyle that you love. It is a plan to lose fat, optimize body composition, build metabolic capacity, and maintain your results for the long term. This plan will require effort, change, and possibly a bit of a learning curve. Nothing worth achieving comes easy. With that being said, this plan will be extremely flexible and sustainable. Once you get the hang of it, there's a good chance you'll fall in love with it.

Calories In

There are two sides to this equation. There're the calories you take in, and the calories that you burn. Let's start with the calories you take in. This section will be a step by step guide for determining what your calorie intake should be for your goal. You will learn how to actually track your calorie intake at the end.

The first thing you will need to determine is your maintenance calories. This is simply the level of calorie intake that equals your caloric expenditure, which would cause no change in body weight. There are two ways to do this: Estimation and trial and error. I recommend a combination of the two; estimating first and then using trial and error to find the exact level. To estimate, you'll simply need your height, weight, age, gender, and probably a calculator.

<u>For men, use the following equation:</u>
66 + (6.2 X weight in pounds) + (12.7 X height in inches) – (6.76 X age in years)

<u>For women, use:</u>
655.1 + (4.35 x weight in pounds) + (4.7 x height in inches) – (4.7 x age in years)

Whatever number you get is a rough estimation of your RMR. Remember that this is only the number of calories you burn at rest. You will now need to make further calculations based on how active you are or how active you plan on being when you start this plan.

There are four activity levels: Sedentary, moderately active, very active, and extremely active. For this, simply use your best judgement and consider how much you exercise, how often you exercise, and how active you are at work. If you sit a desk all day and do two 20-minute sessions of walking per week, you are probably sedentary. On the flip-side, if you work in construction and exercise for two hours every night after work, you are extremely active. Most people will fall between those levels. If you aren't sure, then underestimate.

To calculate, simply take your calculated RMR value and multiply it by the following factor:
Sedentary – RMR x 1.5
Moderate – RMR x 1.75
Very active – RMR x 2.0
Extremely active – RMR x 2.25

Now you have an estimation of how many calories you actually burn every day, which is your maintenance level. This is usually a fairly accurate estimation, but there is a standard error of about +/- 300 calories.

Assuming this estimation is correct, this level of calorie intake would lead to no changes in body weight. So, to set up a proper caloric deficit we have to subtract some calories. One pound of body fat is equal to about 3500 calories. So, a deficit of 500 calories per day would lead to a loss of one pound per week. Many people wonder, how much weight should you try to lose in a week? I would never recommend more than two pounds per week. I consider two pounds per week to be rather aggressive weight loss and certainly not optimal for the long-term unless you have a lot of fat to lose. As a rule of thumb, one pound per week is probably ideal. It is enough to see results quickly and stay motivated, but not too extreme to where hunger and adherence become an issue. If you ever see a headline that says, "lose 12 pounds in 7 days!", just know that the only way to do that is to severely dehydrate yourself and risk your health just to gain it right back.

Even though I consider a 500 calorie/day deficit to be ideal, I don't recommend subtracting 500 calories from your estimated expenditure right from the start. This is because it is only an estimation, and it's better to start with a higher caloric intake and subtract if needed rather than to start too low. I recommend subtracting 200 or 300 to start.

The next thing to determine is the distribution of your protein, carbohydrates, and fats. This simply means the number of grams of each macronutrient you will aim to take in daily. In my view, this is much less important than your overall calorie intake. However, it does your caloric expenditure, and you will want to take in a sufficient amount of each macronutrient to take advantage of their physiological benefits.

The first macronutrient to determine should be protein. For protein, I recommend consuming one gram per pound of body weight. This may seem like a high intake, but protein is very important for reasons that will be discussed in the next chapter. Many people are concerned about consuming too much protein for health reasons. The World Health Organization has found that high protein intake is actually associated with improved kidney function and increased bone density in subjects without pre-existing conditions. Protein, like many other things, has suffered from long-standing myths but is certainly not something to avoid unless otherwise directed by a physician.

Once you have your ideal protein intake, you can determine your intake goals for the two other macronutrients. In order to do this, you must first calculate your calories from protein and subtract this from your overall daily caloric intake. For this step, simply multiply your daily protein grams by four, since there are four calories per gram, and then subtract from your overall calories.

Whatever number you get will be the number of calories you aim to take in from carbohydrates and fats combined. This is where you have some room to adjust numbers based on personal preference. I recommend getting 60% of the remaining calories from carbohydrates and 40% from fats. I make this recommendation for reasons that will be explained in the next chapters. With that being said, diet adherence is the most important factor and if you find that a different ratio suits your preferences better, then by all means adjust those numbers. Just try not to completely avoid either one.

If you choose to go with my recommendation, simply multiple the remaining calories by .6 and divide by four to get your total grams of carbohydrates per day. Then, multiply the same number of remaining calories by .4 and divide by nine to get your total grams of fat per day.

Here is a more visual breakdown of the calculations:

1) RMR formula based on gender
2) RMR X Activity level factor = TDEE
3) TDEE – (200-300 calories) = Beginning calorie intake goal
4) Body weight in pounds = Grams of protein
5) Grams of protein X 4 = Calories from protein
6) Calorie intake goal – Calories from protein = calories from carbohydrates + fats
7) Calories from carbohydrates + fats X .6 = Calories from carbohydrates.
8) Calories from carbohydrates / 4 = Grams of Carbohydrates
9) Calories from carbohydrates + fats X .4 = Calories from fats.
10) Calories from fats / 9 = Grams of fats

An easy way to adjust carbohydrate and fat intake is to remember that you can substitute 25 grams of carbohydrates for 11 grams of fat and your caloric intake will remain the same.

How to Track Calories In

Tracking your food and calorie intake can be tedious at first, but it becomes second nature after a while. There are a lot of useful tools out there these days. I won't recommend a specific brand or app, but just search for "calorie counter" or "calorie tracker" in the app store of whatever smart device you may use. If you don't use one, there are websites that will have most of the same features, and nothing can stop you from using a pen and paper. I recommend the mobile apps because many of the popular ones have a barcode scanner which makes keeping track of packaged items extremely easy. The app or website may ask you for personal information and often a fitness goal as well. They also typically make recommendations for calorie intake goals. Do not follow their guidelines. They are very often inaccurate to the tune of hundreds of calories.

The other item you will want to get your hands on is a food scale. For foods with serving sizes measured in grams or ounces, the food scale will become your best friend. This is especially important for tracking items high in fat. Remember that fat is the most calorically-dense macronutrient. Two tablespoons of peanut butter contain almost as many calories as a cup of oatmeal. You can get away with estimating 4 oz of lean meat or a half cup of rice, but estimating with items like butter, nuts, mayo, and dressings can sabotage all of your effort. I'm not saying you should avoid them, simply make sure you are extra careful with measuring and tracking.

Common items like fruit or eggs can be found in the database of most tracking apps. These you can just search for. However, I generally recommend searching for brand specific entries or using the barcode scanner. Similar items may have completely different numbers for different brands and its important to be as accurate as possible. If you scan an item, make sure you enter the correct serving size or the correct number of servings. With that being said, I also recommend adding individual ingredients rather than a general item. For example, if you are attempting to track a PB&J sandwich, I would recommend measuring the peanut butter and adding it individually, followed by scanning the barcode for the bread and jelly. If you simply search for a generic PB&J sandwich your entry could by off by a few hundred calories. Some bread slices contain 35 calories, some contain 200. Some entries may include one tablespoon of peanut butter, some may include four and it probably won't specify. Again, it all depends on the brand and their recipe.

If you plan on consuming alcohol, your best bet is to stick to light beer or wine. Generally speaking, one serving of each is about 100 calories. To track alcohol consumption, simply substitute it with either your carbohydrate or fat calories. To do this, you should consume either 25 less grams of carbohydrates or 11 less grams of fat for each serving of alcohol.

Calories Out

Now that we've covered how to calculate and track your calorie intake goal, let's talk about how to maximize the calories that you burn on a daily basis. Recall that there are four major components of your daily caloric expenditure: Resting metabolic rate, non-exercise activity, exercise, and the thermic effect of food. Believe it or not, all four of the components can be modified or manipulated. One of the most common mistakes people make while dieting is to simply focus on exercise. Exercise is extremely important, but it's certainly not the only variable.

Let's begin with your resting metabolic rate, since it is the largest component. RMR is largely determined by genetics, which can't be changed. However, there are two additional factors that can be changed which have a substantial impact. Those factors are your body composition, and the severity of your dieting habits. Your body mass has a large influence on the calories you burn. This is why your weight is one of the main factors in the equation to estimate RMR. Every cell in your body needs energy. Muscle mass requires more energy to maintain than fat mass, meaning if you have more muscle you will burn more calories at rest.

This is one of the reasons you will want to maintain as much muscle as possible while losing fat. The severity of your dieting habits can influence your RMR through a process called *adaptive thermogenesis.* This process simply means that there is an additional decrease in metabolic rate, which cannot be explained through a loss of body mass, associated with extreme caloric restriction. This is one of the reasons that crash diets do not work. You will lose metabolically active tissue, but your body will also decrease energy expenditure even further to protect against starvation. Therefore, to maintain a high RMR you will want to maintain as much muscle as possible and only restrict caloric intake moderately. This will be covered in greater depth in the chapter on execution.

Next is the thermic effect of food. Recall that this is the energy required to break down food. The best way to increase TEF is to eat a diet high in both protein and fiber. Relative to the number of calories they contain, protein and fiber both have a TEF of about 30%. On the other hand, fat and non-fiber carbohydrates only have a 3% and 7% TEF respectively. Protein is therefore important for maximizing the percentage of weight lost from fat, for maintaining muscle mass, and for increasing TEF. In order to consume a lot of fiber, I recommend eating most of your carbohydrates from whole grains, fruits, and vegetables. This is also one of the reasons I recommend getting 60% of your non-protein calories from carbohydrates. If you eat a high percentage of carbohydrates, you will likely consume more fiber depending on food choices.

The next component is NEAT, which again is non-exercise activity. NEAT is actually a bit more complex than it seems. It is extremely adaptable. Because it encompasses involuntary movements such as blinking and fidgeting, your body will naturally decrease NEAT when in a calorie deficit. You may not notice it, but you will talk slower, you will blink less, and you will fidget less. Some research has shown a decrease from NEAT as much as 500 calories per day in subjects that were dieting. The only way to combat the involuntary portion of NEAT is to increase voluntary movement portion. You can do this by simply becoming more active in your daily activities. Park at the far end of the parking lot. Stand instead of sitting. Walk during your lunch break. Anything you can think of to move more throughout your day will help.

Last but not least is exercise. I have touched on the importance of resistance training for maintaining muscle and how that indirectly burns calories. However, resistance training also directly burns a large number of calories simply by requiring large muscle groups to use a lot of energy. In fact, it typically burns much more than cardiovascular exercise. I recommend using resistance training as your basis for your exercise routine, and then using moderate amount of cardiovascular exercise as a tool to burn additional calories throughout the week.

There are a million variables to account for with exercise. Exercise should be a stress reliver, not an added source. The biggest variable that will impact results is whether or not you actually get in the gym and put in effort consistently. This will account for 95% of your results. Factors such as the exercises you do, the body-part split you choose, or rep range you work in are all less important details. They certainly have an impact. You should periodically manipulate one of those variables to keep progressing in the gym. I recommend choosing a variable to improve, sticking to it for 4-6 weeks, and then choosing another variable. This could be the weight that you use, the number of reps, the number of sets, or the type of exercise. With that being said, you shouldn't stress out about what exactly to do in the gym. There are a ton of exercise myths and just like with diets, there is no magic formula.

Chapter 6: Execution

Up until this point, you've learned the most important concepts and guidelines. Now it's time to learn exactly how to execute this plan. I recommend using the first week to get an accurate starting point, and to get in the habit of weighing yourself every day. I have witnessed far too many people get frustrated with daily fluctuations in fluid retention. Your weight loss will not be linear. From now on, you are a long-term investor watching a stock price. You know that the price is going to go up and down on a daily basis, but that doesn't matter because you only care about the overall trend of the price. You should apply that mentality to your body weight.

Throughout this process you should be weighing yourself at the same time every single day, and then taking the average at the end of the week. If your average weight is on a downward trend, you will know you're doing something right. From here on out, your goal is to get as close to your numbers as possible. Shoot for the 80/20 rule, which is to get 80% of your calories from foods that you would consider to be "healthy", and 20% from foods that you enjoy. Do this on a daily basis. This process should not be restrictive. Try not go above your calories, but also try not to go below. Remember, you did all of those calculations for a reason. The best way to lose fat is to lose it slowly by maintaining a small calorie deficit over time. Consider it the fat loss sweet-spot. You want your calorie intake to be low enough to burn fat but high enough to maintain your metabolic rate. Your metabolism will adapt to lower calorie intake over time. This is where crash diets go wrong. They are simply too low. A diet is not just one set of guidelines from start to finish. Your body will make physiological adaptations, and you have to combat them. Test out your first calorie deficit. If you find that you are losing an average of a pound a week, you're in the right spot. If you're losing more, then the deficit is too big, and you should add in some calories. If you aren't losing, then you will have to drop your intake.

Most people will see their first plateau within 3-6 weeks. Once this happens, you have to either drop your calorie intake or increase your energy expenditure, usually through more cardio. This is why I suggested only subtracting 200-300 calories for your first deficit. The biggest mistake people make is starting too low and not leaving themselves any room to overcome plateaus. This is absolutely crucial. The process of adaptive thermogenesis will be greater the lower your calories are to start, and you want your metabolism to stay unchanged for as long as possible. For this reason, I actually recommend doing minimal or even no cardiovascular exercise to start out. Of course, it has numerous health benefits and would never recommend avoiding it long-term. However, for this process I want cardio to be a weapon in your arsenal, and I don't want you to use it until you have to.

You'll know you've hit a plateau when you go two or more consecutive weeks without a change in average body weight. At this point, simply subtract 200-300 more calories from your daily intake (not from protein) or add in a few 25-minute cardio sessions per week. I would recommend not doing both, because chances are you will plateau again. This time, you can choose the other option. This way, if you have a relatively large amount of body fat you want to lose, you can alternate between decreasing calories and increasing cardio and go months without making any drastic changes.

This is essentially the entire process; Simply maintaining a moderate deficit and adjusting as you encounter plateaus. It's very simple, but you can see why commercial diets and fad diets don't work in the long-run. They don't consider individual energy needs. They don't account for adaptive thermogenesis. They often start with calories far too low and only give one guideline from the beginning to end. Worst of all, they are often far too restrictive to follow. This plan is inherently less restrictive because there isn't a food item you can't eat. Even still, you will fall off the tracks and accidently eat more calories than you should. In this situation, simply account for it and get back on the tracks. If you go over by 500 calories one day, then all you did was eat your maintenance calories. You can simply write that day off as a neutral day. If you go over by 1000, then simply make up for the difference using the other days of the week. Your hunger will fluctuate on a daily basis and you can adjust your calories with it so long as the average is a moderate deficit for the week.

Chapter 7: Set Point Theory and Reverse Diets

So, here's something that most diet books don't cover: what exactly do you do when you've reached your goal? How do you go about ending a diet? Do you just start eating however you want?

Statistically speaking, the United States actually doesn't have a weight loss problem. The vast majority of people who are overweight will lose a significant portion of that weight at some point in their life. The problem is, over 60% of those people gain that weight back *plus more* within a year. Even worse, after 3 years that number jumps to 95%. The problem is not losing weight, it's losing weight the right way and keeping it off. The way you approach coming out of a calorie deficit can have a huge impact on your long-term success. If you want to keep your results, it must be handled properly. The best way to do this is to use a reverse diet. A reverse diet is simply a gradual, calculated increase in calorie intake that allows for a rebound in metabolic rate and can build your metabolic capacity. If, in the last few weeks of your diet, you were still losing about one pound per week, then you can start the reverse diet by adding back in 500 calories per day. This will bring you back up to maintenance, and you shouldn't gain any weight. From here, the increase should be very gradual. I recommend adding in no more than 100 calories to your daily intake every week. As you increase your calorie intake and come out of your deficit, you may actually need less protein. You can keep it at the same level in grams, and your protein intake will just make up a smaller percentage of your overall calories. Your body won't need to use the amino acids for gluconeogenesis, and it will be more likely to use the protein for remodeling and rebuilding of muscle. To start adding in calories, I recommend increasing your daily fat and carbohydrate intake (in grams) by 2-5% every week. You will have to be pretty meticulous with your tracking, but it's worth it. As you add in calories, your metabolic rate will adapt. Your maintenance calories will actually increase over time. This means that you can maintain your results on higher and higher calories. The next time you diet, you'll be able to do it on higher calories as well. Your BMR, TEF, NEAT, and EAT will all increase. It's even possible to continue to lose fat during this process, if your metabolic rate rebounds faster than your increase in calories. You may certainly notice that you actually continue to look better as you start to eat more. However, this will only happen from a very slow and calculated increase in calorie intake. Everybody is different. Some people may be able to add in 200 daily calories per week, some people may only be able to handle 50 daily calories. Listen to your body and see how your weight changes.

If you properly utilize a reverse diet, you will eventually reach the point where it becomes time for a maintenance phase. A maintenance phase just means you stop adding in calories and you try to maintain your weight for as long as you wish. There are two ways to know when it's time to switch to a maintenance goal. The first way is when you simply reach a level of food intake that you're comfortable with. The second way is when you begin to reach the metabolic "ceiling" and your metabolism no longer responds the same way to increased calories. You'll know when this happens because you'll start to gain weight much more consistently and the changes will be greater. You will gain weight as you reverse diet. The goal is to minimize the amount. As your metabolic rate continues to adapt, your changes in weight may be a bit sporadic. You might gain one week, lose the next, stay the same for a couple weeks, then gain again. This is normal. It's when you start to gain consistently in significant amounts that tells you it's time to back off.

Yo-Yo Diets

Aside from the benefits that come with reverse diets, you'll want to incorporate them in order to avoid yo-yo dieting. Yo-yo dieting refers to the constant back and forth cycle that occurs when you lose weight too quickly, fall off the track, gain it back quickly, try to lose it again, and so forth. This cycle can have very negative effects on the body that many people may not be aware of. Theoretically, your body has a natural range of body fat that it tends to stay in. This range is called your "set point". It is protected by hormonal responses that can change your hunger signals and metabolic rate. As you lose fat, your fat cells shrink and secrete lower amounts of certain hormones. These hormones are what effect metabolism and hunger. So, as you lose fat, you tend to get hungrier and your metabolic rate slows down. As you gain fat, you tend to get less hungry and your metabolic rate speeds up. This is your body's way of trying to keep you in that range. You already know that decreasing and increasing calories has an effect on metabolic rate over time. The important distinction here is that the set point range refers to the range of the body's preferential *size* of the fat cells. Typically, the body only makes new fat cells when somebody becomes very obese. This process is called *pre-adipocyte differentiation*. However, new research has suggested that after a period of caloric restriction, when metabolic rate has been slowed, a large influx of calories can actually cause the same process to occur, resulting in new fat cells. From there, the body still has mechanisms in place to try to return to its preferred *size* of fat cells. Only this time, there will be a higher number of cells than before, and this means a higher level of overall body fat. This suggests that yo-yo dieting and restrictive dieting that results in binging can actually make you fatter over time. This reinforces the fact that long-term sustainable diets are a much better option and that proper reverse dieting is extremely important.

Diet Breaks

There is also some exciting new research on diet breaks, and they may be one of the best tools in your arsenal. Have you ever heard someone say that cheat days help you lose fat because they boost your metabolism? Well, not so much. I find that people approach "cheat days" by just taking the day off and eating whatever they want. Going over your calories one day per week just negates the deficit from the rest of the week. But that idea is on the right track. What the research has found is that taking periodic diet breaks can improve the percentage of weight lost from fat, increase the total amount of fat lost, preserve more muscle mass, and keep metabolic rate sustained better than continuous dieting. The key is that diet breaks do not mean you can eat whatever you want or at whatever calorie level you want. Rather, you must eat at your maintenance level of calories. So, if you're eating at a 500-calorie deficit for a few weeks, you would take a diet break by adding 500 calories/day back in for a week or two. This can be done periodically as another way to combat plateaus and to give yourself a mental break from food restriction. A break should last either one or two weeks. This is a tool not many people use, but it is certainly worth a try. Just make sure that you do it correctly so that you don't end up negating any progress you've made.

Regardless of the method you choose, or how you structure your diet, or what point you're at in your fitness journey, just remember that a long-term approach will always be more successful. Stay mindful of your energy needs, but don't give up if you fall of the tracks. I have seen this method work with people who struggled with traditional dieting for years. Stick to the plan, but don't give up the things you enjoy.

Chapter 8: Final thoughts

The goal of this book was to be different than most of the other fitness books out there. Far too often, people are told what specific foods to eat or when to eat them or how to lose weight quickly for some special occasion that's three weeks away. I see a lot of advice that often does more harm than good. I know how confusing the world of fitness can be, and I hope this book may have shed some light on topics, cleared up some confusion, and given you some new knowledge. As someone who has spent years enduring the learning curve in an extremely frustrating way, I know what it's like. I urge you to email my personal account at DanielMccFitness@gmail.com if you have any further questions. Good luck.

www.ingramcontent.com/pod-product-compliance
Lightning Source LLC
Chambersburg PA
CBHW051126250726
48655CB00007B/2908